Chronic headache and facial pain sufferers experience a silent segregation from the world around them. Their plight is often invisible to the outside world, save those who would read their pain.

From mild to severe, occasional to relentless, symptoms vary widely from one person to another. Often patients have sought answers far and wide. There now exists an accurate method to determine, in a large number of cases, the *cause* of such pain -- cases previously undiagnosed by the Medical and Dental professions. Today's ability to *non-invasively* and *quickly* determine the *source* of the pain in these cases often allows professionals to deliver *predictable,* almost *immediate relief.*

To the "future chronic sufferer," who today has only early signs, yet *no symptoms*, I hope the information to follow will help you comprehend the scope of things to come *before* you realize that "hindsight is 20:20."

This booklet is dedicated to my mother, who has endured chronic leg pain for which medicine has found no cure. I wish that a similar system of diagnosis and predictable relief from her pain might one day be found.

Dr. Tom Orent

INDEX

Foreword 1

1) Headaches and facial pain... a dental problem? And does *dental insurance cover it?* 5

2) How could problems with the teeth cause head & neck pain? 8

3) The anatomy of pain sites in TMJ.............16

4) "But I've never had *any* pain or other symptoms"...18

5) "Could *I* have TMJ?" A 60 second self-screening examination 20

6) Stages of TMJ degeneration:
   a) Early stages of TMJ derangement... "Doctor, I've noticed clicking in my joint, and occasionally...".. 22

   b) Mid-stage TMJ derangements... "Doctor, the clicking has quieted down, but I often wake up with headaches, sore or tired jaws, and 22

   c) Late stage TMJ derangements and the associated severe, potentially debilitating symptoms 25

7) Layers of pain 27

8) "How do I know I should have a TMJ evaluation, and what's involved in the visit?" 28

9) Methods of corrective treatment:

    Occlusal Splint Therapy: "But I've worn *niteguards* before and they really didn't seem to help"...... 38

    The Precision Bite Adjustment 39

    Restorative treatment 40

    Orthodontic treatment..................... 40

    Orthognathic treatment.................... 40

    Combination therapy 41

10) *You* can lead a predictably comfortable healthy, happy life if you are one of many whose pain is associated with joint and bite problems 42

Glossary 43

About the Author 47

❶ HEADACHES and FACIAL PAIN... COULD THEY BE CAUSED BY a *DENTAL* PROBLEM?

Chronic headache and facial pain can range from being occasionally distracting to totally debilitating. Some sufferers have said that others cannot readily imagine their plight without having experienced it personally. Those whose symptoms are mild and infrequent may not even question the source. Others, who've lived with the ongoing battle, may **wonder if they'll ever find long-term relief**. What *is* the source?

Could it be a *dental* problem? A large number of cases involving headache, muscle spasms and jaw joint pain *are* **absolutely a dental problem.** The Medical and Dental professions increasingly are becoming aware of the intricate relationship between proper bite and the muscles and nerves of the jaw joint. A very delicate and predictably reproduceable balance must occur in the chewing system for total harmony, comfort, and stability.

For a large number of patients with facial pain and headaches, the problem and its solution revolve around one of the most complex joints in the body -- the Temporomandibular Joint (TMJoint). The condition is referred to as **Temporomandibular Joint Syndrome,** or **TMJ.** It is not a disease:

it is a simultaneous occurrence of a number of problems associated with the jawbone, nerves, and chewing muscles.

For decades, Medicine and Dentistry have overlooked the Temporomandibular Joint as a potential source of problems. With today's new technologies and increased understanding, dentists with specific, advanced training in TMJ disorders can diagnose and **successfully treat the large majority** of these cases: in fact, if a TMJ disorder is determined, predictable long-term relief is achievable 95% of the time -- via a wide range of *dental* treatments. For long-term relief, TMJ treatments **address the cause of the imbalance** and subsequent pain, **rather than just treat the symptoms.**

For example, here at the Center for Esthetic Dentistry, new team member, Lisa -- who worked full-time for eight years for various dentists -- suffered from severe headaches six out of seven mornings. We found a cause-and-effect relationship between the way that her teeth met and functioned, and her chronic pain. Even in the earliest stages of treatment, **within the first 24 hours, she was pain free**.

Physicians also have a recently heightened awareness of the relationship between facial and headache pain and the Temporomandibular Joint. Another case concerned a patient who, even taking two Percodans at a time, had been in the acute phase of pain, for weeks, with no relief. We performed a simple test that confirmed our suspicions -- the cause-and-effect relationship between her bite, the nerves and muscles of the jaw joint -- and her pain was identified. During this brief evaluation, we also commenced a temporary treatment that afforded her **predictable, total relief within hours!**

About DENTAL INSURANCE: Dental Insurance companies have but a single goal -- show the highest profit to their shareholders and directors at the end of the fiscal year. As long as employers keep buying their plans (*income*) and the insurance companies minimize benefits paid (*expenses*), they will prosper. Since it is extremely difficult for employers to understand all the terms and conditions of the plans they purchase for their employees, bottom line costs are usually the primary consideration.

Dental Insurance companies may **deny benefits for your treatment by categorizing TMJ Syndrome as a medical condition.** This maneuver is truly a "Catch 22": **you may be reimbursed if you receive** *medical treatment* for what is now **scientifically proven** to be **treatable 95% of the time through** *only dental* **means!**

Occasionally, they may reimburse physical therapy, including ultrasound treatments and/or TENS (transcutaneous electronic nerve stimulation). Is there merit to this "*medical*" treatment? Absolutely. *However,* in **95% of TMJ cases, medical treatment alone is severely limited, as it addresses only the symptoms and not the cause.** Any relief afforded is temporary, at best.

② HOW COULD PROBLEMS WITH THE TEETH CAUSE HEAD AND NECK PAIN?

TMJ Syndrome is a simultaneous occurrence of a number of problems associated with the jawbone, nerve network and chewing muscles. Once you understand why your body does what it does, together we can use that knowledge to correct the cause of the problem -- not just treat symptoms.

The Nerve Network:
At greater than 20,000 cell endings per square millimeter, the dentin, or inner tooth structure, is one of the most sensitive and *perceptive* parts of the human body! If you've ever bitten down on a few grains of sand in seafood, you've experienced the awesome sensitivity of the system.

Working in conjunction with the nerves of the dentin is the extremely sensitive network of the periodontal ligaments. Teeth are attached to their bone sockets by thousands upon thousands of tiny fibers called periodontal ligaments (PDL), each with its own nerve and blood supply. If you've had a few fibers of floss caught in your teeth -- and it felt like a brick was stuck in between -- you've experienced the PDL nerves in action.

These neural networks constantly update your brain about your teeth, much as air traffic controllers use sophisticated radar systems to three-dimensionally locate planes. They carry information about position and contact, and they can sense the *tiniest* contact imaginable!

The Temporomandibular Joint:
The **TMJoint is one of the most complex joints in the body.** Not only does it work like a hinge, allowing the initial opening and closing of your mouth, but the entire system can slide forward and down the skull. Try these movements: open and close your mouth without allowing your tongue to leave the roof of your mouth, and you'll feel the "hinge action" of the joint. Now, allow your lower jaw to swing as far open as possible, as in a yawn. The latter half of that motion is a sliding action, during which rotation may also occur.

The **TMJoint includes a critically important little disc** -- the intra-articular disc -- which keeps the top of the jawbone from direct contact with its bony socket in the skull. Both sides of the disc are constantly bathed in one of the most slippery lubricating fluids known to man. This disc has the difficult job of keeping pace with the actions and sliding of the jaw during opening and closing. If the jaw is only hinging, the disc moves about only slightly. When the jaw's sliding mechanism comes into play (e.g., when you open wide to bite a sandwich, or to yawn), the disc must rapidly travel with the jawbone.

The disc itself is merely cartilage, and has no nerve endings; it bears all the forces of chewing in total comfort. The front of the disc is held and controlled by a muscle called the lateral pterygoid, and the back of the disc is held by ligament fibers.

Part of the lateral pterygoid muscle, which guides the disc, is responsible for opening and pulling the jaw forward, right and left: it is quite adept at its job.

The Chewing Muscles:
The **muscles** of chewing span from the temples to the bottom of the jaw, forward to the cheekbones. They are **programmed for a precise and beautiful coordination**: the muscles that close or "chomp" down are very powerful, while the opening muscles are more delicate.

Picture your front teeth touching together, edge to edge, as if to incise off a piece of thread. Imagine if your brain allowed your full set of closing muscles to go into action, and close with the power reserved usually for chewing straight down on the back teeth! If you try this, you'll find your body will not allow you to close down with any force, except when the back teeth are ready to come together.

When your jaw closes and the teeth clamp straight down, the full force and strength of the closing muscles is unleashed. But as soon as your teeth move in *any* other direction (side to side, or toward the front), the back teeth *should* come slightly out of contact with each other, and the powerful closing muscles *should* immediately shut down.

A Problem:
Muscle incoordination occurs if and when any back teeth

touch while the jaw is forward or chewing side to side. As soon as any premolar or molar contact occurs, the dentin and periodontal neural networks signal the brain, which instructs

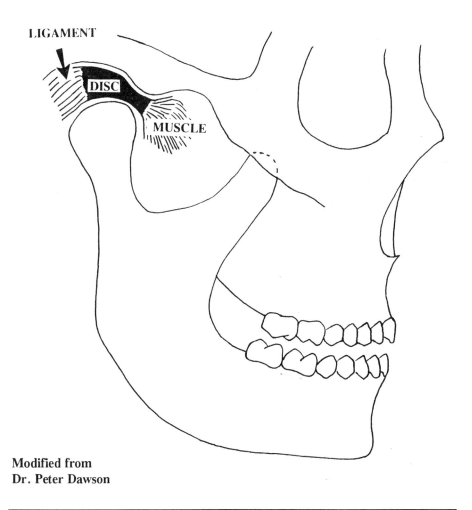

Modified from
Dr. Peter Dawson

Normal alignment of the disc within the joint

the powerful chewing muscles to clamp down. But the jaw is not centered to close straight down on the back teeth! The lateral pterygoid muscle, fully aware, "fires" to try to shift the jaw right or left, in an attempt to "go around" the spot that shouldn't be allowed to hit! This spot is called an **"interference."**

When one has even the slightest improper contacts or *"interferences,"* the lateral pterygoid muscle will fire -- all day long! Every time we chew, every time we swallow, in fact every time our teeth touch. **The muscle becomes hyperactive, and the pain begins.** Like in any other overworked muscle in the body, lactic acid builds up; the muscle can't get enough oxygen to wash it away, and the pain cycle commences.

Not only is the lateral pyterygoid muscle painful from constant hyperactivity (overuse), it is equally sore from the "antagonistic workout" it gets when fighting the closing muscles, which kicked in when a back tooth came into contact. Try making a muscle with your biceps by pulling your clenched fist up toward your shoulder. Now have a friend pull the fist back away from the shoulder while you try hard to oppose his action. This type of **antagonistic, spastic muscle incoordination is at the heart of the chronic pain experienced with TMJ problems.**

A comfortable position for your joint, and a **comfortable place for your bite** must occur simultaneously. Muscle harmony, jaw joint and teeth stability and comfort *depend* on this relationship.

The most comfortable position for any joint is within its normal range of motion. Once pulled forward or forced even slightly out of joint, the associated muscle groups will be signaled into action.

If you've ever had a filling or other type of dental restoration placed, you already know the most comfortable position for your bite. Immediately after placement of a new restoration, your dentist checks for "high" spots; until they are eliminated, the bite is extremely uncomfortable. The most comfortable place for your bite allows simultaneous, even contact of all teeth.

The majority of patients with Temporomandibular Joint (TMJ) Syndrome exhibit a discrepancy between the comfortable position of the jaw joint and that of their teeth. That is, the teeth cannot all meet simultaneously when the jaw joint is within its normal range and hinged closed. Typically, one of the back teeth hits first. The incredibly sensitive nerve system recognizes the premature contact, and calls for the powerful closing muscles to continue their contraction until the majority of teeth are in contact. The lower jaw pivots about the tooth in premature contact. The top of the jawbone pulls down away from the skull, as the front lower teeth rise up toward contact.

Once the teeth reach *their* comfortable destination, the joint complex is significantly stressed. Muscle hyperactivity occurs for several reasons: first, the lateral pterygoid fires in an effort to *avoid* the interfering contacts, instantaneously

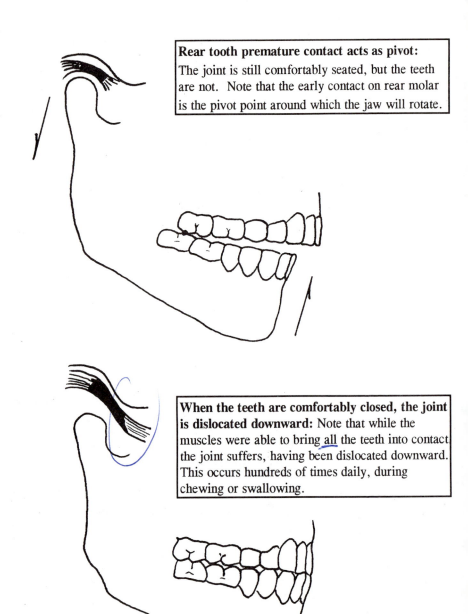

Modified from
Dr. Peter Dawson

shifting the jaw imperceptibly to the right or left based upon its memory of the contact.

Second is the stretch receptor reflex. Tendons attach muscle to bone; when the jaw joint is stressed (or dislocated), the tendons' stretch receptors become activated. They signal the brain that a potential injury is in progress.

The third source of muscle hyperactivity occurs once the teeth contact comfortably. Now the jawbone is stretched down from *its* comfortable position, and the closing muscles fire by reflex.

Most **TMJ treatment is focused on harmonizing a comfortable bite while the jaw joint, too, is in its comfortably seated position.**

THE ANATOMY OF PAIN SITES IN TMJ

Another source of pain occurs when the intra-articular disc is unable to do its job properly. The lateral pterygoid muscle is responsible for guiding the disc forward. In cases of hyperactivity it may pull the disc forward so that the disc slips in front of the jawbone -- even when the jaw joint is not in its forward sliding mode. When you open your mouth, the jawbone "pops" back onto the disc, which is waiting out in front. This is the "click" or "pop" some patients experience.

The ligament attached to the back of the disc is very sensitive, making it **a potentially severe source of pain**. Unlike the disc's cartilage, ligaments have many nerves and blood vessels, which cause severe pain if compressed. When the disc is forward, the top of the jawbone sends chewing forces against this sensitive retrodiscal ligament. Some patients suffer severe pain when chewing or yawning, for example.

The jaw joints are immediately in front of each ear. The muscles for chewing span from the temple to the bottom of the jaw, forward to the cheekbone. Understanding human anatomy makes it is easy to comprehend how **hyperactivity, followed by lactic acid build-up in muscles of the jaw joint, could cause significant facial pain and headaches.**

Stress was once thought to be the cause of TMJ disorders. Our current understanding classifies stress as *one* contributing factor, but certainly *not the cause*.

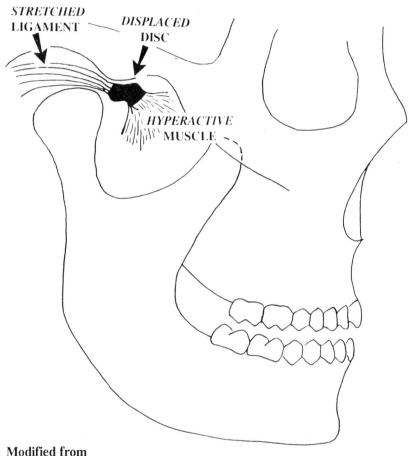

Modified from
Dr. Peter Dawson

Disc displaced forward of the joint

"BUT I'VE NEVER HAD *ANY* PAIN OR OTHER SYMPTOMS..."

Today, we have advanced diagnostics in many areas of Medicine that afford us forewarning of problems to come. For example, a simple blood test can tell us of **cholesterol levels today**, which may lead to **tomorrow's stroke or heart attack.** Similarly, routine screening mammography today can prevent the heartache of undetected untreatable cancer tomorrow.

Severe consequences can be avoided with *proactive diagnostics* and *preventive* intervention. Ninety-five percent of TMJ problems are caused by an imbalance in the relationship between the teeth, muscles, nerves and jaw joint. Similar to the silent problems mentioned above, **TMJ problems, left untreated, lead to degeneration of bone, muscle, ligaments, or all three.**

Eventually one or more of the following is possible:
* Limited range of motion of the jaw (such as the inability to open wide enough, even to brush properly);
* Severe pain when chewing;
* Frequent episodes of grinding, extreme muscle tension and constant head, neck, and facial pain;
* Severe (destructive) premature, abnormal teeth wear.

Early treatment is easier, faster, less costly and more

predictable than ever. The longer you wait, the more complex the degeneration and less predictably stable the outcome of treatment. We cannot predict the pace of degeneration nor the possible eventual level of derangement or dysfunction for any given individual. But, predictable long-term correction is highly likely for those patients fortunate enough to **identify a TMJ disorder** *before* the degeneration is allowed to **decrease their quality of life**. We *can* achieve a harmonious, peaceful and balanced masticatory system.

⑤
"COULD *I* HAVE a TMJ PROBLEM?"
A 60 SECOND SELF-SCREENING EXAM

Temporomandibular Joint Syndrome is *not* a disease. It is a simultaneous occurrence of a number of problems associated with the jaw joint, nerves, and chewing muscles.

A "screening history" can be worthwhile whether you have symptoms, or not. **For those with absolutely no symptoms, the screening can be especially helpful:** only by such means can we proactively identify and minimize future degenerative problems. **Patients suffering from chronic severe pain and headaches also can benefit greatly** from the screening: a positive result may signify the first step toward reduction or elimination of chronic pain.

See next page for self-screening quiz.

PLEASE TAKE A MOMENT TO COMPLETE THE FOLLOWING SCREENING EXAM:

Comfortable resting place

- ❏ Have you *ever* heard any clicking or popping in your jaw joints (immediately in front of your ears)?
- ❏ Have you ever experienced headaches, near your temples, upon awakening in the morning?
- ❏ Have you ever experienced chewing muscle soreness or tension upon awakening in the morning?
- ☒ Have you ever had jaw joint pain during chewing? *Rarely*
- ❏ Has yawning or opening wide ever caused you pain?
- ❏ Has your jaw ever been stuck or locked open, even if only for a brief moment?
- ❏ Have you ever felt that your teeth didn't meet in a comfortable position?
- ❏ Has a dentist ever devoted one or more appointments to precision bite adjustment or "equilibration?"
- ❏ Have you ever been struck on, or received traumatic injury to the head, neck or jaw? *Left side of skull*
- ❏ Have you ever had any episodes of pain in the jaw joint?
- ☒ Have you ever ground your teeth while sleeping?
- ❏ Do you find yourself clenching your teeth during the day?
- ☒ Do your jaw muscles tire while eating or talking?
- ❏ Do you have Arthritis?
- ☒ Have you ever been treated in the past for TMJ problems?
- ❏ Have you ever noticed: difficulty or limitation in opening? Or,
    - ...recent shifting, crowding, rotating or new spaces opening?
    - ...or, loose teeth?

Although some questions carry more weight than others, a thorough **TMJ Evaluation** should be performed if there are **three or four positive answers** to this quiz.

⑥
STAGES OF TMJ DEGENERATION

A) Early Stage TMJ Derangement: "Doctor, I've noticed clicking in my jaw joint, and occasionally..."

In the early stages, patients with Temporomandibular Joint (TMJ) problems may **not experience obvious symptoms,** save an occasional faint click, for example. The disc is just beginning to intermittently slip forward of the jaw joint, and in almost every case, there are problems -- though imperceptible to the patient -- with the teeth. Yet, it is *possible* to experience symptoms (occasional grinding or clenching, slight muscle soreness, an occasional muscle tension headache, etc.) for which TMJ is *not necessarily* the culprit.

Cases treated in this early stage have the highest probability of *complete* recovery and long-term stability, especially if treatment is commenced within one year of onset. Treatment is often less involved, and there is a very high success rate. Unfortunately, treatment may be delayed because symptoms are often minimal or absent in this stage. Most cases **successfully** diagnosed and **treated** in the **early stages** were **detected during a screening history session.**

B) Mid-Stage TMJ Derangements... "Doctor, the clicking has quieted down, but I often wake up with

headaches, sore or tired jaws, and..."

"Middle-stage" is comprised of a wide range of degenerative problems associated with TMJ disorders. Patients may have experienced numerous symptoms (see Self Screening Exam, Chapter 5), or relatively few, ranging from mild and sporadic to chronic and severe.

It is **human nature to take a "wait and see" attitude** when we first experience seemingly minor insignificant symptoms, especially those associated with a potential TMJ disorder. **Many TMJ symptoms can be confused with other relatively harmless maladies** including (but not limited to) sinus, tension or migraine headaches, minor tooth irritation, occasional ringing in the ear, and the shifting or wearing down of teeth incorrectly attributed to the "natural aging process," among others.

The "wait and see" philosophy can be prolonged by the usual physiological course that TMJoint degeneration manifests. Many patients assume that the click is harmless, and forget about it entirely when it goes away. But, TMJ disorders classically follow a degenerative pattern, frequently including a history of a click that disappears over time. Remember -- in the early stages, the intra-articular disc intermittently slips off the jaw joint. The click typically represents the jaw joint slipping back *on* to the disc upon opening, and then back *off* during closure. At this stage, the disc is intermittently displaced forward of the joint space.

Although clicking often can be heard in serious mid-stage

problems, it also can have disappeared at this point, as well. The **history of a click for a period of time, followed by cessation of that click, without intervention, often indicates the next and more serious level of joint degeneration.** At this point, the disc has been displaced and totally locked out forward, no longer allowing the jaw joint to slip on and off during function.

This means any time pressure is placed on the joint (biting, chewing, etc.) without proper alignment of the intra-articular disc to bear the forces, potentially mild to severe pain ensues as the jawbone presses on the sensitive retrodiscal ligaments. Plus, a self-protective mechanism of the body causes excessive grinding and clenching in an effort to "erase" the interfering surfaces of imbalanced teeth. The effort is not only futile, but accelerates the degeneration of the entire masticatory system.

In other words, tooth enamel wears at an abnormal rate. In some cases, that wear progresses right through the enamel into the yellower inner tooth layer called the dentin. Unfortunately, the dentin is not only a far more sensitive structure, it **is 7 times softer than tooth enamel.** The resultant destruction can rapidly destroy the remaining natural teeth.

As tooth wear accelerates, muscle hyperactivity worsens, often accompanied by pain caused by pressure on the retrodiscal ligament. Patients in this middle stage also may experience limited ability to open (due to muscle pain and spasm), and abnormally rapid fatigue of the jaw muscles while chewing tough foods or gum, or even talking for an extended period of time.

Middle stage derangements classically exhibit such a wide range and varied combination of signs and symptoms that the only accurate assessment is through proper jaw joint examination and bite analysis. Proper diagnosis of TMJ problems is dependent upon a complete and thorough examination by a dentist who has specific, advanced TMJ disorder diagnosis and treatment training (see Chapter 8).

C.) Late Stage TMJ Derangement… "Doctor, I've had chronic headaches for quite some time, which nobody has been able to solve. Recently I've also experienced difficulty in chewing and even opening my mouth as widely as I used to…"

When treated in time, **95% of TMJ** disorders are **predictably correctable without surgical intervention**. It is my sincere wish that this booklet will help potential sufferers long before they reach the latter stages.

In advanced joint disorders, some patients experience moderate to severe chronic pain. But for others, the pain has totally ceased.

Sadly, the cessation of long-term chronic pain is most likely indicative of a complete and irreversible perforation of the ligament that holds the rear of the intra-articular disc. Subsequently, the **patient's ability to open and chew may**

be severely limited, and will likely continue to worsen for the remainder of his or her life. Although pain caused by pressure on the retrodiscal ligaments is gone, patients may still suffer from headaches and muscle spasm. At this stage, treatment is aimed at minimizing the structural degeneration of the jaw joint itself, and maximizing patient comfort.

In advanced cases -- where the disc is locked out forward, and the jawbone has completely perforated the retrodiscal ligament -- subsequent bone-to-bone contact occurs. The **head of the jawbone now rests directly against the skull** without the protective advantage of the highly lubricated intra-articular disc. The **bone continues to break down**, shortening the height of the rear portion of the jaw. As the jaw's length diminishes, the patient's rear-most teeth enter into abnormally excessive contact; they require grinding, by the dentist, to enable complete closure of the teeth without jaw joint displacement. Grinding will likely be necessary once or twice annually for life. Patients with this stage derangement should be aware of the need for ongoing adjustments, the possibility of limited jaw opening, and potential necessity for rear-most teeth extraction.

LAYERS of PAIN

A high percentage of patients who pursue the diagnosis of chronic headache and/or facial pain have only one major source of pain. In those instances, the diagnosis *and* treatment are usually straightforward.

Others may suffer from TMJ pain, plus pain from one or more additional sources, simultaneously. For example, migraine headaches, although *not caused* by TMJ problems, *may be triggered* by tooth-muscle-joint imbalances. Other pain sources may include (but would certainly not be limited to) systemic diseases, cancer, fibromyalgia, etc.. Although multiple layers of pain may exist, we are still able to isolate, identify and, in most instances, correct problems associated with the jaw joint.

⑧
"HOW DO I KNOW I SHOULD HAVE A TMJ EVALUATION? and WHAT'S INVOLVED?"

The recommendation to undergo a TMJ evaluation should be made by a dentist with training in the diagnosis and treatment of TMJ problems. *However,* the simple screening test (see Chapter 5) is often sufficient to alert patients to the need. If you have positive answers for three or four of the screening questions, an evaluation would be prudent.

The evaluation will vary from patient to patient, depending upon the suspected severity of degeneration. It may also vary among practitioners, depending upon their training and their available equipment. The most expensive testing (e.g., Magnetic Resonance Imaging, or MRI) or surgery is limited to patients exhibiting the most advanced stages. The majority of patients can be accurately diagnosed -- and an effective treatment plans developed -- from the routine evaluation described below:

TMJ Ultrasound: Using technology similar to the Doppler used to monitor the fetal heart, the TMJ Ultrasound (in conjunction with a thorough history) affords us a clear understanding of the stage or level of jaw joint degeneration. It is a *non-invasive,* **painless examination that enables us**

to visualize that which, once, only could be seen with exploratory surgery. The TMJ Ultrasound has a high degree of accuracy and relative low cost.

A normal healthy joint is silent during function. A clicking or popping noise is indicative of intra-articular disc displacement. The click is heard as the disc dislocates in and out of the jaw joint. Based upon the timing of sounds with respect to specific jaw motions, the jaw joint ultrasound can pinpoint which portion of the disc has been displaced.

Whether the disc has been partially displaced or fully locked out, damage to the retrodiscal ligaments can occur. In the absence of the smooth bearing surfaces of the disc, the top of the jawbone rubs against the bottom of the ligaments that tether the rearmost aspect of the disc. This type of abrasive interaction may be asymptomatic in some patients, or a source of great pain for others. The Doppler Ultrasound isolates this damage as a coarse grating sound during functional jaw movements.

Mobility: 95% of TMJ problems are bite-related muscle imbalances: the forces of bite are misdirected on one or more teeth. Inappropriate forces can cause mobility, or **looseness of teeth, often imperceptible to the patient.** Testing for mobility is quick and simple. A sturdy instrument (e.g., the handle of a dental mirror) is placed on one side of the tooth, and the dentist's finger, or a second instrument, is placed on the other side. Gentle pressure exerted from side to side lets the dentist determine the presence or absence of abnormal mobility. The patient often is unaware of any "loose" teeth, and surprised to see demonstrable mobility in teeth caused by the forces of improper bite alignment.

Periodontal Disease Screening: Periodontal disease is most often caused by a bacterial infection of the gum, ligaments and bone that support the teeth. Normal healthy gums have minimal space or opening where the gum edge meets the teeth, a maximum **depth of 2 or 3 millimeters.** Healthy gum does not bleed during a depth measurement evaluation.

As periodontal disease progresses, the bacterial infection causes an acid breakdown of the protective band of gum closely attached to the tooth's root, creating a pocket. The bacteria multiply in their new home, deep in the base of the newly formed pocket.

Here's a good analogy: look at the healthy cuticle of your thumbnail to visualize the process. Although a blunt-ended periodontal probe might sink a millimeter or two between the cuticle and nail, it could not go any further, and the measurement would not cause bleeding. It would be cause for great concern if your thumb were infected to the extent that a probe could drop down 5 or 6 millimeters between the nail and cuticle -- and blood oozed from the site!

Periodontal health is critical because gum disease can damage the bone. Unless eliminated, the **bacterial infection in the periodontal pockets** (5, 6 or more millimeters deep) will begin acid **destruction of the bone.** As the bony tooth socket deteriorates, the tooth become loose and mobility can be measured.

The destructive nature of periodontal disease becomes a vicious, downward spiraling cycle. Improper tooth contacts caused by mobility initiate muscle incoordination and hyperactivity, traumatizing the teeth with excessive force at damaging angles. In some cases, bone damage is caused even without the presence of periodontal infection -- merely from the imbalanced forces of bite.

Bite Analysis on Simulator: Impressions are made and models of your teeth poured in plaster. Although many patients have had impressions taken before, analysis of the bite cannot be performed from the models alone. If you think of the TMJoint as the pivot point for all actions of the jaw, you can see how the spatial relationship (distance and precise location) between the jaw joint and the teeth would change how the teeth meet. If the distance were increased or moved off to one side slightly, all contacting points would be changed.

The precise relationship must be measured, recorded, and transferred onto an "articulator," a laboratory bench top instrument for precise simulation of teeth contact during functional movements. Several relationship measurements will be made, with special non-distortable waxes, allowing a diagnostic quality simulation.

Evaluation of the most comfortable place for your bite versus that for your jaw joint: Almost everyone has a position considered the most comfortable for their teeth to meet. It occurs when the teeth are in their most closed position: i.e., when you chew straight up and down, and then clench tight together, this is the "most closed position." Similarly, like every joint in the body, the jaw joint is most comfortable when fully seated.

If the teeth all meet simultaneously as the jaw joint hinges closed, there is harmony between the teeth, nerves muscles and the joint itself. If, however, *any* tooth contacts *before* the others, a pivot point is established, and disharmony begins. In order to **test for the existence of "premature contacts,"** which **interfere with system harmony**, a special gentle manipulation of your jaw will be performed. During this procedure, your jaw joint will be fully seated, and all muscles relaxed. If an interference or discrepancy exists, it will be readily obvious to both dentist and patient at this point.

Load Testing: Perhaps the most critical test of the jaw joint, the "loading test" measures the ability of the joint to comfortably bear various amounts of pressure. **A healthy TMJoint is able to bear almost any amount of exerted force** without causing pain, tenderness or even tension in the joint muscles. Yet, because of the body's incredible ability to adapt to abnormal conditions and stress, even a jaw joint that has undergone various stages of degeneration usually is able to pass a loading test.

Pain, tenderness or tension in the joint muscles during the loading test is indicative of one of two things: either the jaw joint was not seated fully in its socket, or there is an "Intracapsular Disorder."

The former is usually caused by hyperactive muscles constantly contracting due to disharmony and imbalance. Often, the dentist can resolve this by repositioning the jaw joint and trying again. Or, the dentist may place cotton rolls between the patient's teeth for a sufficient period of time -- enabling the muscles to deprogram (lose their memory of the interfering contacts). Once relaxed, the muscles allow the jaw joint to seat and the loading test should be normal.

If these attempts fail, it could indicate that the muscle memory was too heavily ingrained to be "deprogrammed" in such a short period of inactivity. If this is the case, the patient may have to wear, overnight, a muscle deprogramming device like the Occlusal Splint. The splint is a precision-fit plastic guard that simulates your perfect bite, thus eliminating all interfering contacts. By the next day, the jaw joint will have fully seated because the muscles had the chance to relax.

A failed test also may indicate an "Intracapsular Disorder," which is a level of **jaw joint structural degeneration**. Bite/joint disharmonies, left to deteriorate without proper treatment, can lead to osteoarthritis. This condition is a gradual breakdown of the outer layer of bone at the top of the jawbone. The worse it gets, the more difficult treatment becomes.

Another Intracapsular Disorder is the locking out forward of the intra-articular disc. In this position, the disc is rendered totally ineffective for protecting the health of the jaw joint. If the blood supply to the jaw joint is pinched off --

subsequent to the disc locking out -- a dramatic and traumatic condition known as **Avascular Necrosis (AVN)** can occur. **Patients usually report a sudden loud "pop" near the ear.** At the same time, they may find their bite has instantly changed for the worse -- they may have become unable to touch their front teeth together, for example.

The vast majority of patients pass the loading test with ease. Although passing the test absolutely does not rule out intracapsular joint problems, failing the test (as described above) may indicate the existence of a serious condition.

Muscle Testing: Hyperactivity of the muscles plays a pivotal role in TMJ problems. By simply exerting differing amounts of pressure directly on various chewing muscles, the dentist can ascertain whether or not the muscles have been over-exerted. Normal, **healthy muscles can take various levels of pressure without any discomfort.**

Wear Patterns: As described in Chapter 2, no back teeth (molars or premolars -- i.e., all teeth in back of the canine or "eye-teeth") should ever come in contact except when chewing straight up and down. So, the discovery of any pattern of wear on back teeth is indicative of an imbalanced bite. The back teeth should be unable to contact in any grinding motion (front to back *or* side to side); thus, any flattening out or "wear facets" are abnormal.

Since the body is aware of the potential harm caused by this type of inappropriate contact, it attempts (in futility) to "erase" the offending interfering contacts. The **"erasure** mechanism" is manifested as **teeth grinding or clenching**, an action that, unfortunately, not only is unable to eliminate the offensive contacts, but seriously worsens the overall condition. The major muscles of chewing are activated at a time when the front teeth are at risk, placing undue forces on them.

Unlike most other parts of the body, there is no mechanism for the repair or replacement of tooth enamel. Once the enamel is worn through, the inner dentin is exposed. Dentin is far more sensitive, and **7 times softer than enamel!** Once bite patterns have caused the loss of enamel at a given site, **continued wear, if allowed, will progress 7 times faster than before!**

The result of teeth grinding is hyperactive, often sore-to-the-touch muscles, worn teeth, the creation of new and worse interfering contacts, and often the **degeneration of the Joint-Disc Assembly**. As discussed previously, when the lateral pterygoid muscle is hyperactive, its upper portion can pull the disc forward and off the jawbone. In early stages the jawbone is able to pop back on and off -- producing the "click" described by many patients. In later stages, the disc remains locked out forward and the click is no longer heard.

Guidance Analysis: Chapter 2 discusses the body's intricate system to sense "interferences," inappropriate contact points. When an interference is present, equilibrium is severely compromised because the delicate balance between the muscles, nerves, jaw joint and teeth is destroyed. "Guidance" refers to the mechanism that protects us from interfering contacts and subsequent disharmony.

As we slide our teeth anywhere out of the centered position -- forward, right, or left -- some combination of the canines (eye teeth), and incisors does all the work. These front teeth "guide" the jaw so that the premolars and molars cannot touch. If wear, gum disease, fracture, or decay were to compromise any of these teeth, there is a high likelihood that back tooth contact would be introduced upon lateral or forward chewing. **The unaltered health of the bottom six front teeth is critical to the protection of the long-term health and function of the entire system.**

Proper analysis of effective, protective guidance requires careful observation of *all contacting surfaces* during *all possible chewing movements*. Clinically, this can be accomplished by placing extremely thin foil (8 micron) or colored marking paper between the back teeth during sliding motions. Interferences exist if you can catch the test foil (or mark with the paper) on any premolar or molar (other than when your jaw is centered).

The most accurate analysis requires impressions, or molds of your teeth, from which plaster models are made. Then, very precise wax records are taken. These measurements record the relationship between the joint and the upper jaw, and the jaw-to-jaw relationship when the joint is fully relaxed. This information, in conjunction with the models of your teeth, creates a working simulation of your exact biting motions -- revealing exactly which teeth contact during various movements. With this analysis, **we can determine how best** to perfect a harmonious system that protects the comfort, beauty and longevity of your smile.

Range of Motion Testing: Measurements are taken of the patient's maximum ability to open straight up and down, and side to side. Restricted motion, relative to known averages, most frequently is indicative of muscle hyperactivity. Occasionally, limitation may indicate structural breakdown of the jaw joint itself.

⑨
METHODS of CORRECTIVE TREATMENT

"If a diagnosis of a TMJ disorder is made, what are the possible treatments I could expect?" Careful analysis and diagnosis leads to the most conservative, effective treatments possible. There are six categories of potential *non-surgical* therapies. *Surgical* intervention is required *less than 5%* of the time.

Occlusal Splint Therapy: An occlusal splint is a clear plastic guard that fits over the upper (or occasionally lower) teeth. Although it may look like the common *"niteguard,"* there is a dramatic difference: an occlusal splint will simulate the perfect bite pattern. All teeth will touch with even, simultaneous contact as the jaw moves straight up and down. At the beginning of any grinding motion (toward the front or either side), all of the molars and premolars come out of contact. In the majority of cases, a well-made splint will relieve most or all pain from TMJ muscle hyperactivity -- usually within the first 24 hours.

When would the dentist suggest a splint?

A) When immediate relief is critical. Anyone suffering from acute or chronic TMJ headaches and pain is fully aware of the debilitating nature of their problem. In an emergency, a splint can be constructed and placed in a matter of hours.

B) **Delta-Stage Bruxers.** Although most grinding occurs during lighter stages of sleep, some patients do their most destructive grinding during Delta stage sleep. If grinding continues after reconstruction, or originally was severe enough to extensively wear of the natural teeth, a night splint may be required.

C) **Unable to "Load Test."** Chapter 8 discusses the "Load Test" and its sources as either an Intracapsular Disorder (degenerative structural joint problem) or muscle hyperactivity. In most cases, muscle hyperactivity can be relieved sufficiently by the splint to allow normal load testing. If still unable to load, further diagnostics may be required, including TMJ x-rays and/or MRI (Magnetic Resonance Imaging).

Although splints are extremely effective, they are usually an adjunct or precursor to proper bite rehabilitation. If the involved teeth are not treated properly, the cycle of excessive wear, muscle hyperactivity, spasm, pain and eventual jaw joint degeneration will continue.

The Precision Bite Adjustment (PBA): The Precision Bite Adjustment (or "equilibration") is the simplest and most conservative method of perfecting the bite to eliminate the interferences. PBA is the selected option when the dentist determines that removing the interfering contacts will not appreciably compromise the anatomy of the teeth, and will not remove enamel to the extent that dentin is exposed. Often, analysis of the bite simulation models (see Chapter 8) helps determine the extent of adjustment necessary .

The PBA usually requires two or more appointments, with the first as much as an hour long; sufficient time is required to perfect the bite during every functional movement of the jaw. Rather than creating a "new bite," we are only re-enabling what once was. An anesthetic is not required, as the amounts of tooth structure removed are minimal -- similar to adjusting a high spot on a filling, with the drill.

Restorative Treatment: Restorative treatment consists of procedures normally performed to rebuild broken, decayed or missing tooth structure (or teeth), such as onlays, crowns, bridges or partials. Because the stability of the newly perfected bite and patient's health are compromised by older fillings with broken or leaky edges, decay or fracture, these may be removed during the restorative process.

Orthodontic Treatment: It may not be possible to perfect your bite with Precision Bite Adjustment (PBA) and/or selective, restorative treatment. Occasionally, one or more teeth may not be able to achieve a stable position without first being slightly moved. Orthodontics, in many instances, may be limited to "minor tooth movement." A simple removable retainer, or a temporarily bonded wire or rubber band may be used to gently move the tooth in question. Only in *severe* cases of malalignment would full braces be considered.

Orthognathic Treatment: Although rare, there are situations that necessitate moving a segment of bone along with the teeth. In these unusual cases, growth and development have not allowed for proper facial configuration: the size and shape of the jaws do not adequately match the teeth. In these *rare* cases, surgical intervention is required for proper realignment.

Combination Therapy: In most instances, some combination of the above treatments is employed. Most frequently, Precision Bite Adjustment is performed along with necessary restorative care.

More severe cases require combinations of treatments, as well. Skeletal developmental problems, as well as traumatic accidents, may require combination therapy that could span the entire spectrum of care.

⑩
YOU CAN LEAD a PREDICTABLY COMFORTABLE HEALTHY HAPPY LIFE

It is my hope that a better understanding of anatomy and TMJ syndrome will encourage those who have yet to experience symptoms to undertake a *proactive* course of action. Remember, considerable damage can occur long before symptoms are enough to cause concern. Hindsight is 20/20: it is my sincere wish that this common degenerative process be halted as early as possible.

For those who already have experienced chronic TMJ-related pain, the predictability of treatment (in greater than 95% of cases) should offer considerable peace of mind. There are definite steps to be taken -- both to properly assess your existing condition, and then choose the most appropriate conservative treatment. Our goal is optimal, maintainable oral health, enabling patients to look and feel good throughout life.

GLOSSARY

Articulator: A laboratory benchmark instrument for precise simulation of teeth contact during functional movements.

AVN: Avascular Necrosis, a dramatic and traumatic condition caused by pinched-off blood supply to the jaw joint. The top of the jaw bone eventually implodes-- like an empty eggshell being crushed in.

Click: The sound made when the jaw bone positions itself back onto the intra-articular disc, which has been dislocated forward, in front of the jaw bone.

Dentin: The yellower inner tooth layer, 7 times softer than tooth enamel and far more sensitive. Dentin wear progresses 7 times faster than tooth enamel, and cannot be repaired or replaced by the body.

Erasure Mechanism: The body's automatic and futile attempt to rid interfering contact by teeth grinding and jaw clenching.

Hyperactive Muscle: An overworked muscle that does not receive enough oxygenated blood flow to keep pace and counteract lactic acid build-up.

Interference: Improper tooth contact preventing maximum simultaneous tooth contacts while the joint is still fully seated.

Intra-articular Disc: A cartilaginous disc that floats between the top of the jaw bone and its bony socket in the skull, one on each side of the head. Bathed in a slippery fluid, the disc eases the actions and sliding of the jaw. A healthy, properly aligned disc can withstand even the greatest forces of chewing without the slightest discomfort.

Intracapsular Disorder: Jaw joint structural degeneration, in which there is a gradual breakdown of the ligaments and/or bone at the top of the jawbone-- often characterized by long-term dislocation of the intra-articular disc.

Lactic Acid: A normal byproduct of worked muscles, an overload of which causes muscle pain.

Lateral Pterygoid Muscle: Holds and controls the front of the intra-articular disc; responsible for opening and pulling the jaw forward, right and left.

Load Test: Measures the ability of the jaw joint to comfortably bear varying amounts of pressure.

Masticatory System: The muscles, nerves, TM Joints, jaws and teeth which work together to enable chewing.

Mobility: Looseness of teeth, often imperceptible, frequently caused by the forces of improper bite alignment.

Muscle Incoordination: Condition which occurs when back teeth touch during forward or side to side chewing. Normally, back teeth should not touch while the jaw is in these positions.

Occlusal Splint: A clear, plastic guard that simulates the perfect bite pattern.

Orthodontic Treatment: Methods of enabling tooth movement, ranging from simple retainers and rubber bands to bonded wires and braces.

Orthognathic Treatment: Surgical procedure used in rare cases to correct the size, shape, and/or alignment of the jaws

PBA: Precision Bite Adjustment (also called *equilibration*), a conservative method of perfecting the bite by removing small amounts of tooth structure with a dental drill.

PDL: Periodontal Ligament, a tiny fiber with its own nerve and blood supply. Thousands of PDLs attach each tooth to its bone socket.

Periodontal Disease: Bacterial infection of the gum, ligaments and bone that support the teeth.

Premature Contact: Condition in which any tooth touches before the others, creating a pivot point and dislocating the jaw joint as the remaining teeth come together.

Restorative Treatments: Procedures normally performed to rebuild broken, decayed or missing tooth structure, such as fillings, crowns, onlays, implants, and bridges.

Retrodiscal Ligament: Ligament fibers which hold the back of the intra-articular disc.

TMJ: Temporomandibular Joint, or the jaw joint.

TMJ Syndrome: A Simultaneous occurrence of a number of problems associated with the jaw joint, nerves, teeth, and chewing muscles.

About the Author

Dr. Tom Orent lectures to dentists internationally on Reconstructive Dentistry. He has been a guest lecturer at The University of Nevada, Las Vegas, New York University, and Tufts University School of Dental Medicine. He has served as a member the faculty at Boston University School of Graduate Dentistry, and as the editor of the *Journal of the American Academy of Cosmetic Dentistry*.

Dr. Orent has served on the ethics committee of the AACD as well as the accreditation review board. He is the President of the New England Chapter. Dr. Orent maintains a multi-specialty private practice of reconstructive and cosmetic dentistry in Framingham, Massachusetts, the Center for Esthetic Dentistry (508-872-0045).

- → large number, majority
- → Why not all, which issues can't be addressed

I do have more headaches

Facebow

Myopractic Adjusment → leveler and ogy

- Don't know how to hold jaw
- Can't find resting place
- Headaches more frequent
- Molars on right side hit first
- Slight Overbite?!?
- Weak Muscles always needing to be adjusted

→ Need some re-assurance/guarantee on Splint/Appliance

Where am I - As far as severity

TMJ Ultrasound - Used here?!?

How loose are my teeth

Ceramic/Heat Treated neutral filling a 10

P-10 by 3M a 1

What's in between